Empowered | Pain-Free

EmmaSara McMillion CNHC

Fearless Childbirth

Copyright 2018 EmmaSara McMillion

Unless otherwise indicated, all Scripture is taken from the English Standard Version (ESV). The Holy Bible, English Standard Version. ESV® Permanent Text Edition® (2016). Copyright © 2001 by Crossway Bibles, a publishing ministry of Good News Publishers.

New King James Version (NKJV). Scripture taken from the New King James Version®. Copyright © 1982 by Thomas Nelson. Used by permission. All rights reserved. King James Version (KJV). Public Domain.

ISBN -13: 978-1725769731

Editor: Bijou McMillion

Formatting by– Nile McMillion

Illustrator- Davae McMillion

Compelled Lifestyle Publishing

PO BOX 1043

Alpine, TX 79831

Dedication

This book is dedicated to every woman who has ever given birth, whether natural or C-section, at home or in a hospital, with pain meds or without.

It is also dedicated to every woman who has endured troublesome childbirth. May this book bring you hope and encouragement.

Acknowledgments

Thank you to my daughters who were by my side to provide comfort and support through so many of my deliveries.

To my husband, Clinton, thank you for growing with me in the discovery of positive birthing.

Finally, to my future legacy of grandchildren. I pray this book launches a thousand ships of supernatural birth experiences for generations to come!

A Note For You

This book was written out of my heart's desire to help labor become a better experience for every woman.

Better is better, and a beautiful delivery is to be sought after with hope. May you find encouragement through the pages of this book.

EmmaSara McMillion

Mama of 8 blessings

Table of Contents

Preface

The Birth Experience

Every woman who has ever given birth has her own story to share. Personally, I have eight stories, and I feel that it is safe to say I know the difference between painfully severe versus positive-empowered labor. Out of those eight deliveries, six of them were excruciating and let's just say, I will spare the details. There are enough birth horror stories floating around. My intent for this book is to bring hope to those who have fears about labor and delivery. Think about it, if childbirth was easy and joyful, instead of full of fear and anguish, how would that impact women today? Wouldn't moms-to-be feel encouraged about the birthing process? How would the hope of a joyful birth impact you?

You are probably reading this book because you have questions. One question might be, "Is it even possible to experience pain-free childbirth?" Maybe you are wondering, "What would a positive, intentional childbirth even look like?" If either of those questions hit the spot, you are not alone. I had those same questions, and they consumed me for nine months before my last baby was born. As a pregnant woman carrying my eighth baby to term, my desire was to have a trauma-free labor and birth experience. I know there were some people who hid their laughs at my high hopes as if I were convoluted. That's fine, I understand there are always going to be skeptics in the house. I mean, how unrealistic can someone be to think that's even possible, right? The truth is, just a few pregnancies ago I didn't think it was possible and until just recently, I think I would have called it very hopeful. I had no problem stating that children are a blessing, but not so much for childbirth. With all honesty, it felt more like a curse than a blessing in my moments of agony.

However, today I know it is possible! Why? Because I did it! I had an intentional, positive, trauma-free childbirth experience with no excruciating pain!

I can now say that childbirth is indeed a blessing! Do you want to hear some exciting news? It only took a couple of weeks before my baby was born to prepare my mind for intentional childbirth! It was enough time to give me the tools to achieve total control during labor. What do I mean by total control? I wrote this social media post the day after my delivery, describing the beautiful feeling of empowerment I felt while in labor.

"A baby wasn't just born yesterday, but also another level of trust and commitment in my marriage. I know my husband saw a side of me that he has never seen before. How do I know? Because I conquered something for myself. #TotalControl I have never been able to pull it off to such a degree before... Complete control of my being, emotions, person, fears, and ideas. I chose

truth and faith... I give thanks to Yahweh for strengthening me every step of the way."

Total control defined for me is being in complete control of my person and most importantly, my mind. By making a lot of little decisions, I kept calm. My midwife pointed out that I was constantly working with, instead of against my body. I believe this is part of what produced such a positive experience for me. I can't wait to share my testimony with you so you can glean insight to have your own beautiful story to share. The contents of this book are my answer to many prayers for a smooth birth.

My prayer is that pregnant mamas who read this book will also get to have a "me too" phenomenal birth story to share. How wonderful would that be?

Chapter 1

Re-education

At the age of twenty-five, I gave birth to my first child in 1999 in the basement of the hospital in Chania, Greece. Since I was a first-time mother, I had no idea that some of their practices could be considered rough and dangerous. It was a fast and hyped up three-hour labor experience that I won't soon forget! Just under two years later I delivered again, but this time I had my son in a stateside hospital with a midwife. My labor was five hours long, and I can remember having time to ponder life as I listened to soulful praise music. It was a very spiritual experience for me. As I had contractions, I can remember thinking of Christ on the cross and the pain He endured for my sins. I felt connected in His sufferings and to be honest I felt the weight of my many sins as if I should be suffering in childbirth. As crazy as this might sound, I felt a level of guilt, and at the same time, like the pain felt right. Like I deserved to be suffering. Recently, I found that CD from previous labors that contained worship songs that focused on reaching out to God in times of trouble. My first son was brought into the world to the sound of Amazing Grace playing in the background. After such a hard time in the basement in Chania, this labor seemed so much "nicer" even though I experienced some real pain during my contractions. For the next six deliveries, I focused on the same area of scripture that spoke of childbirth pains (aka sorrows) increasing because of Eve's fall. -Ref. Gen. 3:16

Since I was stuck on that passage, I was blinded. I could not view the act of childbirth as a blessing. After each child, labor felt more and more like a curse which led to more fears. Fast forward to 2014, where I found out that I was pregnant with my seventh child. I was excited that I would have a new bundle to love, but I wasn't feeling the excitement of yet another labor. Gratefully, a friend of mine could sense my inner turmoil, so she dropped off a book for me. That was a real game changer! It was *Supernatural Childbirth* by Jackie Mize. The focus of the book was about experiencing the promises of God concerning conception and delivery, and as I began to read, I had a deep revelation. I realized that I had an improper view of the full work that was done and completed for me on the cross of Calvary. As a believer, my understanding was clearly skewed! However, I intend to stick to the heart of the matter rather than to try and present a theological dissertation for you. Basically, I realized I kept identifying with the suffering of the account of Genesis instead of the redemptive work of Yeshua/Jesus.

Galatians chapter 3 states that we have been redeemed from the curse! That means the penalty of sin has been paid in full! There are so many scriptures that support this truth. How did I miss this? I don't have a clear answer for you because I do love to read my Bible. However, one thing I feel is certain is that Christ redeemed us from the curse of the fall in Genesis.

"Christ hath redeemed us from the curse of the law, being made a curse for us: for it is written, cursed is everyone that hangs on a tree." -Gal 3:13

After my understanding was enlightened, it permitted me to believe in the finished work of Christ. Now I was excited and had hope for a better way to labor! No longer was I expecting to suffer. Instead, I was looking forward to experiencing great joy!

"Lo, children are an heritage of the LORD: and the fruit of the womb is his reward." Psalms 127:3-5

If the fruit of the womb is a reward, I thought to myself, then I will stand and proclaim that birth should also be a reward! Not too many months after I read Jackie's book, I gave birth to my precious seventh child. I went into the birthing center filled with peace and hope. I am sure you are all wondering how that turned out. Well, it turned out much better than any of my other six experiences. I went up to the later stages of labor without any great pain. I felt like everything was bearable until the pushing portion arose. The battle for the mind was on! I almost conquered it, but a moment of fear came in and with it so did pain. It was only for about ten minutes, but it was enough to cause me to question if I could do it again. Fast forward three years to now...

Going into the eighth round of having another child, I was determined to completely push back fear! **The determination to do hard things is beautiful when you can persevere!** What was so neat about it was that it felt so right and calm, despite a tiring pushing session. It was so simple, it just wasn't easy. There was still work involved. What do I mean by that?

Think about a marathon. The concept of the race is simple but participating in it isn't easy. If it was, there wouldn't be such a feeling of great accomplishment when you crossed the finish line. On the day I delivered my baby I felt like a triathlete that accomplished much because I did! I finished tired and sweating, but victorious!

Chapter 2

Standard vs Natural Process

"Throughout the last and current century, two different birth philosophies have existed in the United States. The most prominent of these is the medical management model. This framework starts with the premise that pregnancy and birth are intrinsically difficult and potentially dangerous processes that when left to occur naturally, frequently result in poor outcomes." This model has taken birth from a natural process in most women's lives to a medicalized procedure similar to one of disease management, with multiple interventions." -National Library of Medicine

In my pursuit of a new way to labor, I had to confront old mindsets. In one breath I spoke negatively about the medical community's philosophy of child birthing, but in the next breath, I agreed with it by sharing my horror birth stories with others as if experiencing pain was the only way. I bought into the lie, then I went and perpetuated it!

Let's face it sometimes it is hard to deal with the facts. If you've had multiple tough labors, it could be difficult to convince you that it is meant to be joyful and trauma-free. To some, it may sound absurd or too good to be true. However, there is a whole movement that thinks differently. There are those who are spreading the positive birth message internationally.

"A positive birth means a birth in which a woman feels she has freedom of choice, access to accurate information, and that she is in control, powerful and respected. A birth that she approaches, perhaps with some trepidation, but without fear or dread, and that she then goes on to enjoy, and later remember with warmth and pride." Positive BirthMovement.org

It has been noted that most women who use positive birthing methods do not feel labor "pains," but instead feel a pressure that is mitigated or decreased with deep breathing and relaxing thoughts. Traditionally most women experience **FTP**, a **Fear-Tension-Pain** cycle during birth.

Fear= Believing lies, remembering past pain, doubt and not trusting your body.

Tension= Resistance, anxiety and emotional trauma, leading to slow down, exhaustion and regression.

Pain= Possible intervention, baby distress, and less oxygen.

Wouldn't a better solution be to replace F.T.P. with **C.R.P.E.**?

Confidence.
Relaxation.
Peaceful.
Empowerment.

I love the thought of "**peaceful empowerment**," because it reminds me of the verse, *"In quietness and in confidence shall be your strength."*- Isa 30:15

Just after I had the baby that scripture came to mind and I realized that the battle of the mind is won with quietness and confidence. By adopting a "shalom mindset," you are choosing peace. When we choose peace, it helps invite oxytocin into our labor process. Oxytocin is the baby bliss hormone.

When you have a positive birthing experience the amount of oxytocin that floods the body truly produces a natural high like no other. After labor, I was very exhausted, but that didn't stop the flood of empowerment that swept through my body post labor! After I had a snack, I seriously felt like superwoman! For a moment in time, I was a birthing champ! I felt such a sense of accomplishment and gratification. I felt like, what couldn't I conquer after squashing so many fears about labor?

Positive birthing has been shown to produce: easier, shorter labor, more efficient progress, less intervention, fewer pain meds, more positive experiences, fully present mothers, and calmer newborns. I can attest to the calmer newborns. My longest labor was also my hardest and was traumatic, and my newborn was a wreck. He was highly emotional, very sensitive to sound and he had a nervous belly. My two positive birth babies were so notably calm, and both did great their first night with me.

Of course, there are no guarantees of outcomes. **Each birth story is unique**, and the addition of medical interventions can create an environment where the body is being asked to do things it is not ready to do. Gratefully, I didn't have to have any medical interventions which allowed for nice progress. However, results may differ. I spent the past three years doing a mind overhaul for other areas of life which helped me in this area. I guess you can say, I was primed to take every thought captive and for the process of believing and receiving. This book was born out of my desire to share information with you, so that you can make informed choices that could enable you to remain in control during labor.

My suggestions given are for educational purposes only and are taken from personal experience. They are not intended as medical advice. Pregnancy is a journey that is very personal. I hope this book helps you find peace and fulfillment on your path.

Chapter 3

My Pain-Free Birth Story

When I found out I was pregnant this time, I decided to believe for a delivery free of excruciating-pain. I was so confident about my decision that I didn't go into an in-depth pursuit of tools until the end of my pregnancy! I did still have Jackie Mize's *Supernatural Childbirth* book. However, life was packed for most of my pregnancy, so I didn't pick it up again until I was about thirty-six weeks pregnant. I just skimmed through it, and I felt confident that I understood the message loud and clear. As a matter of fact, you can see my relaxed thinking in the following social media post written in my 3rd trimester:

"I will be 36 weeks prego this week! Boy, this pregnancy is different than my other pregnancies. Once, I actually had a baby shower at nine weeks pregnant! Really!

If you are wondering why I had it so early, it's because I lived in Greece and it was the only time I was going to be stateside. Now, here I am with the baby most likely engaged. He is low and knocking daily on my belly as if to tell me he is ready to see the world and I don't have much prepared. Clinton told me days ago, "Hun, get things ready." However, I haven't done much to get ready yet because space is so limited, and I had to take the time to try and clear out some stuff from our room that is shared with his five brothers' clothing too. Before I did some packing, I found myself googling checklists as if I am some rookie! Today I was so tired, and Clinton walked in and saw me on the bed and said, "There she is, still is." I just couldn't get my body moving."

Although I felt healthy in the final weeks of my pregnancy, I was exhausted. One week after that post, my family took our RV/home and drove three hours to the city to be near my midwife. I went in for my appointment that day, and I was effaced 2cm. There were no other notable changes in ripening. That was a little surprising since I was so stinking sore down yonder! My last baby was fully "engaged" weeks before also, but I didn't remember being so super sore. I can only describe it as a bruised feeling. Since I hadn't seen much progress, I decided to do as much walking as I could before my due date, which unfortunately caused even more soreness as you would expect. But I figured I could walk and get things moving since he was so low, or I could lay in bed every day and slow down the process. I decided I'd rather do some walking. A few days after getting settled in at an RV park, I started doing some positive birthing research.

At this point, I had heard about supernatural childbirth, but not the positive birthing community. I wasn't sure what to think about it, but it piqued my interest. As I started to research, I definitely found some things that intrigued me, yet there were others that I didn't feel comfortable with. So, I decided to approach it the way I have with integrative health. I have been researching integrative holistic medicine for fifteen years, and many of the modes of health I lean towards are Ancient Eastern protocols. I believe in viewing a person entirely mind-body-spirit, rather than just looking at symptoms as isolated. I have studied eastern medicine that focuses highly on digestion and herbs for health. However, I separated ideas that did not fit my convictions, yet I received full benefits from practice insights. I came to the same conclusion when contrasting *supernatural childbirth* with the *positive childbirth community.*

I found that Supernatural childbirth methods seemed to rely solely on faith, but there were many women who tried it yet-did not have the experience they were hoping for. Dare I say, they lacked faith? Who wants to tack that onto a disappointing labor experience? As I watched many different positive birthing videos, I noticed one common thread between them. It was more about relaxation, focus, and being educated on how the body works during labor. In contrast, the supernatural labor stories, faith alone, either worked or it didn't.

I started to wonder if there was more preparation besides faith that I could enter labor with to give me a better opportunity to have a successful experience. I definitely didn't think it had to be one way or the other. So, I concluded that I would still stand upon my principals of faith and adopt the positive affirmation portion of what positive birthing had to offer along with pursuing a better understanding of my body during labor.

I feel that those two areas lineup with my belief that words are powerful and have the power to bless and curse. I also believe that knowledge is power and understanding of the birthing process would allow me to premeditate what to expect with a new mindset and without fear. Many birthing sites I visited practiced standard hypnotism, and I was not interested in being hypnotized. Instead, I am into being in control of my person which is why I never took any kind of drugs for any of my seven other deliveries. Being totally present and aware of my surroundings was and is very important to me. However, I found helpful hypnobirthing sites that were not about being hypnotized at all. Instead, the content was created to have mom-to-be totally focused on the moment with a positive mindset. So, three weeks before I gave birth, I submerged myself in gleaning all I could on how to have a beautiful childbirth experience. I focused on the promises of God and filling my mind with positive words about childbirth. I learned proper breathing exercises. I was educated about the body's basic workings during labor and how to submit to the process. Basically, I went through a re-education of the labor process, and I graduated on my delivery day!

Now on to my birth story!

The day of my delivery I did this social media post:

Post 2/14 (Day of delivery)

Yesterday just after 2 p.m. my cervix and membranes were swept. Afterward, we decided to go for a two-mile walk to get things moving and I also did some breast pumping. I have been extremely sore because this baby's head has been low, low, as in my DOWN LOW region for weeks! It feels like I am walking with a melon between my legs and like I just rode in a rodeo! However, I didn't let that stop me from walking. It was a great day with the kids. As of yesterday, I was 3 cm. Today February 14th, earlier I was 4cm, and 5/6 cm stretched which spells progress! Can you please pray against fear because **faith and fear are opposite?** *Pray against it at any point in my labor. Pray, I will focus on TRUTH and not lies which produce greater faith which = Supernatural Childbirth.*

I am currently at 7 cm with zero pain! Pray for a quick delivery because my midwife just broke my water!"

My birth timeline rundown began at 2:30 p.m. on Feb 13th when I had my membranes swept and then I went for a family walk. It was so amazing because we were walking through a neighborhood when suddenly one of my sons pointed to the street sign and said, "look, a sign!" I was so surprised! There was my baby's name (which isn't common) on a street sign! You know we got a photo below it! It felt like it was a sign from heaven that the baby was drawing near.

That evening we stayed in the birth center in case things got rolling quickly. I was super sore, and it was even hard for me to walk. Thankfully I was allowed access to the large tub, so I took a nice warm herbal bath with some essential oils in it while I had my diffuser with rosemary going. It was so wonderful and tranquil. I also had strong surges (aka contractions) that were notable, but I didn't bother trying to log them because I was at the birthing center. I could just hear the words of my midwife ringing in my ear, "You are safe here. Just get as much sleep as you can." In the past, the beginning of contractions could have thrown me overboard, but instead, I was listening to my affirmation audio all night and doing my up breathing that was very relaxing. My contractions or what I called surges were strong enough to momentarily wake me, but not strong enough to keep me awake. I felt very calm and excited that my baby was going to be coming soon! I felt in control.

The next day, February 14th, I woke up at 8 a.m. with continual surges that felt productive but were very sporadic and spaced apart. I could honestly barely walk. I had to get around with an ice-skating motion because my groin was too sore to lift my legs. If I did it hurt, but it was not a labor pain. About 1 pm I decided to try the bouncing ball. Typically, I loathed the bouncing ball during my past labors. But I told my husband that I wanted to try it again because I had a new mindset. "Let's give it a go!" I sat down, and what do you know, I liked it!

My midwife then came in and had me use the breast pump. Looking back, I had the machine turned up too high because my boobs were very sore before the baby was born which impacted nursing.

At **2:45 p.m.** my midwife broke my water. Shortly afterward, my husband asked if I could take a nap which the midwife allowed, so I took an hour nap. Around 3:45 p.m. I started to walk around in the birthing center and not long after my surges began to get more frequent and intense, but completely manageable. Remember at **2:30** I was already at 7 cm without even knowing I progressed so far.

At **4:51 p.m.** I felt a slight urge to push, and my midwife confirmed I was at 10 cm without doing an internal which was a relief. So, I started some breathing exercises and tried some pushing. I was in need of a perk up because I was feeling tired, so I asked for my cloth with rosemary essential oil on it. It brought such comfort when I would smell it. A bit later I remember feeling a little queasy, so I asked for my peppermint cloth to whiff, and that completely took care of that issue. It was just amazing that I went to 10 cm without pain. It all happened pretty fast, but I was still tired from all the lack of sleep the weeks before. Plus, I got up a ton of times to go to the bathroom the night before every time I had a surge.

At **5 p.m.** the pushing urge subsided some. I was resting my head on my pillow as I was kneeling and hanging over the side bed. My legs were getting weary, and on top of that, I was doing my breathing wrong for pushing. Oh, the things we learn. At **5:50 p.m.** the strong urge came back and more focused pushing began. I pushed off and on for 15 minutes before my legs felt like noodles because I was kneeling on them as I was hanging on the side of the bed. I thought maybe I overdid myself the day before with my two-mile walk! So, I asked to be moved to the birthing chair which interested me. I had never tried it before, but it kept wooing me to sit on it to give my legs a rest. I should mention that now that I have tried other positions for childbirth if given a choice I would not choose to lay on my back to give birth. Gravity is your friend when giving birth and laying on your back can slow transition down.

Finally, at **5:55 p.m.** I moved to the birthing chair, and it was such a relief. It felt soft and comfortable. I leaned back on it and tried to push, but I kept pushing wrong which was delaying the process. I also realize now that I was reclining too much! I kept forgetting to push my breath down far enough. At one point my midwife told me, "get angry at it EmmaSara!" In the past, I was very efficient at pushing because I was filled with adrenaline and fear. "Fight or flight" would kick in, and the process would go much faster. However, this time there was no surge of adrenaline, so things were slower, but they were not painful. I was tired and exhausted! I felt like I was doing an Ironman competition and I was nearing the finish line. I was just trying to muster up the energy to complete the race. I can remember defeated thoughts trying to swim into my mind, but just as soon as they came in I would swipe them right out! You know those thoughts, "What if I don't have enough energy to finish? What if we encouraged birth too soon?" They would pop in and then I would swipe them right out!

At **6:34 p.m.** I remembered one of the midwives telling me the only issue she has seen with positive birthing methods is that a mom would be so relaxed that she wouldn't feel such a strong urge to push. It was at that moment that I decided to stop lounging on the birthing chair and asked to be moved back to the bedside. I also asked for my leisure affirmation audio to be changed to a powerful praise song that I was listening to earlier during latent labor. My midwife chimed in and asked for it to be turned up louder! Also, instead of hanging extended over the edge of the bed I leaned back on knees away from it as if I was going to go potty. I can remember telling myself, "You are a last inning girl! You are a grinder! You can do this!"

At that moment at **6:37 p.m.,** just 3 minutes after changing my position and changing my mindset- I gave a perfect deep inward down breath, I felt the baby literally drop, slide down and crown! I actually smiled at that point!

Success! Finally, I was about to see my baby! My midwife told me to slow down, and I remembered that the time had come to "breathe" my baby out. I was so calm, and it happened so fast. I felt the baby's head pop out, but it was unusual because normally someone calls out that the head is out, but no one said anything. Later I was told they (my family) didn't say anything because they didn't know it happened! They said by the look on my face they had no idea that I just pushed the baby's head out! Once the baby was at his shoulders, the midwife asked my husband if he was going to catch the baby because he was already halfway out. My husband was shocked and lunged forward to catch him. I did it! I conquered my fears and conquered pain!

I trusted God and my body, and at 6:41pm February 14, 2018, my baby was born free of trauma and I did not feel excruciating labor pains! There were some obvious uncomfortable times and it was with a great effort for sure. I was super exhausted before my labor ever began or I am sure it would have even been easier had I not been so tired and sore down yonder! I would describe my transition as intense, and I really had to work on pushing because I was so relaxed, but it was all manageable. Did you hear that? Yes, manageable. In the past pushing was something like torture and this time it felt so rewarding afterward like I just crossed a finish line, tired, sore, out of breath, yet TRIUMPHANT!

Chapter 4

Understanding Your Body

Fear is a silencer. Fear can stop a woman from having a voice and sometimes it can cause women to be closed to knowledge and understanding. I have never had a problem having a voice, but boy was I closed to hearing about the birth process. I felt like listening to or exploring the details of birth would somehow cause even greater pain. I think I felt that if I knew more, it would cause greater turmoil. During one of my labors, I can vividly remember a midwife holding a mirror asking me if I would like to see while I was pushing. I was horrified! No, I didn't want to see that big head pushing through my body! I was holding on to the mentality of "hear no evil, think no evil, speak no evil." So, I went through eight pregnancies avoiding looking into the birthing process in great depth. I think many women feel the same. What is so strange is that I am a woman who is constantly teaching about the topic of empowerment. Not only that, but I am also a lifestyle coach, holistic health educator and so many times I have been a voice for the voiceless. I was also a children's safety advocate and former director of a women's and children's shelter. However, when it came to birth, I felt like my hands were tied and my eyes had a blindfold around them. The worst part was when labor finally came I felt like I had no control over the process. I felt like I was in for a ride that would take me places I wasn't interested in venturing towards.

Fast forward to my twelfth pregnancy and eighth delivery. This time around I was ready to learn and grow because I was ready to conquer fear! After my last labor experience, I had a taste of supernatural labor, and I wanted to run after a full testimony. I watched video after video of women sharing their pain-free experiences, and I set my heart and my mind on having my own story to share. I had to make a conscious decision to conquer my fears head-on. With that decision came some strategic planning.

My strategy was to create an order of education. The order went like this:

1) Watch and listen to only positive birth testimonies free of trauma.

2) Learn labor techniques and about how the body works during the labor process.

3) Study positive birthing affirmations.

4) Watch positive birthing videos.

5) Invite my husband to learn about the birthing partner aspect of labor

6) Listen to affirmation audios nightly and during labor.

This was my recipe for education and empowerment. And, most importantly it was my strategy to conquer my fear of knowing "too much." So, that meant watching babies descend and be pushed out! Previously, I could not watch that part of the process on video because it was attached to too much trauma. Now, here I sat post-strategy smiling and experiencing great joy while watching that section of positive labor videos. If you receive anything at all from this book, I hope you understand that **saying yes to fear is saying yes to pain. If you can say no to fear, you can say no to pain. If you choose to swipe fear away, tension and pain can go away right along with it!** Situations may arise that are out of your control, but there is one thing you **can** control, and that is your response to challenging situations. Remember no matter what arises, you can remain calm. If things start to take a turn from your original plan, don't go into panic or frustration mode. Choose to remain as calm as you can and let negative feelings go for the sake of your delivery. I lean on the fact that fear is not of the Lord and that perfect love casts out all fear. Remember; as you think in your heart so shall you be.

I believe that words are powerful and that we should take every thought captive. I believe that knowledge is power. So, I am extremely

42

interested in the science behind positive birthing. Understanding about inputs and outputs of birth is now fascinating to me. After just a few weeks of researching I found a lot of information on how to have a beautiful birth experience and applied them, and they worked! I admit I felt a little frustrated because I wasn't aware of my options with my other deliveries, but I quickly turned the disappointment into a passion for sharing my findings with anyone who is interested. Children are a blessing, and I want childbirth to feel like a blessing too.

The Science of Positive Childbirth

Science supports the practice of positive childbirth techniques. It also highlights the impact fear has on the body.

Fear Tension Pain Syndrome is a concept by Grantly Dick-Read MD to explain the pain commonly expected in childbirth. He concluded that attitudes are a catalyst for anxiety before labor and cause fear in labor.

He proposes that "**fear causes muscular and psychological tension that interferes with the natural process of dilation and delivery, leading to pain.** He advocated education, exercise and warm emotional and physical support in labor to counteract the syndrome and coined the term natural childbirth for labor and delivery in which the well-trained woman joyfully, comfortably and with a calm, cooperative attitude participates in a natural experience."-Mosby's Medical Dictionary

Normally, he said, birth *is "carried out by natural processes from beginning to end, influenced by natural emotions and perfected by the harmony of the mechanism [with the woman] conscious throughout the progress of her baby's birth, so that she can truly fulfill herself emotionally when she sees and welcomes the child emerging from her womb into the world,"* GD: *Natural Childbirth. London, Heinemann, 1933.*

For too long, traditional medicine has allowed much fear to perpetuate in the minds of women and even some men. However, even if you are birthing in a hospital, you can choose to make it a positive experience by using as many tools as you can to conquer FTP Fear-Tension-Pain syndrome. **Removing fear is the key to experiencing a positive birth. This means permitting yourself to STOP listening to birth horror stories at all cost!**

Transition without FTP

Onto the subject of **transition**. Even if you have a relatively easy latent/active labor experience, the transition could really test your endurance. Even during my transition phase, I was tired. I definitely experienced some huge body shifts. However, I remained focused. I used all my "labor tools," and I was able to get to full dilation and still keep my composure. I even have a photo laughing between surges. The biggest part of my education came when I realized that a woman's body is created to birth beautifully and that our body wants to give life. It is a beautiful process and not one to be feared. Every step-in labor our body is preparing to usher in life. Why would we want to shut down that process after so many months of excitement and anticipation? The answer is because the traditional medical system has taught us that labor is a medical procedure that necessitates intervention and medication many times. **The truth is that if we work with our body, it wants to work with us.** What a revelation! **We can be co-laborers with our body.** We can work with the process instead of against it. When we work together with it, it is like a beautiful duet. We can make beautiful music together. We can strike a chord in the heavenlies. Are you ready to create your personal rhythm and tune?

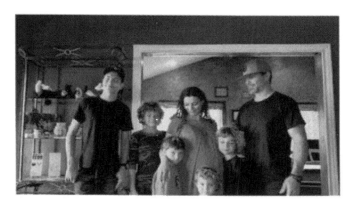

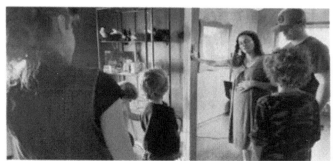

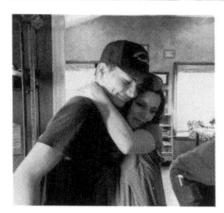

Just before I was ready to push, I spent a few minutes with my male clan...

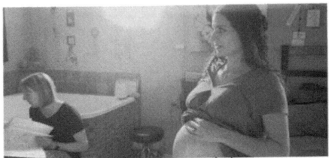

The atmosphere was glorious.

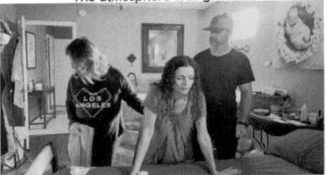

Go time! Time to push.

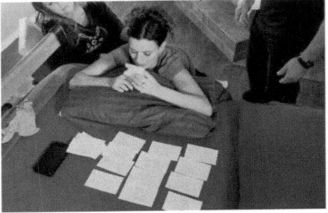

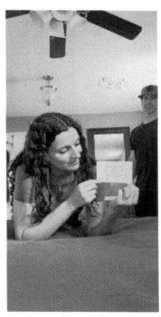

Over 8 cm dilated

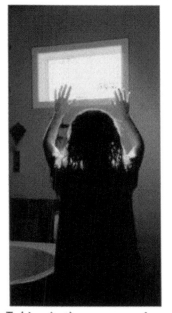

Taking in the sun, praying.

At 7 cm, doing some pelvic tilts

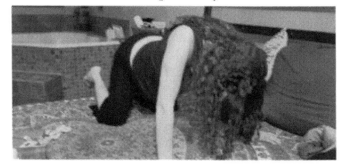

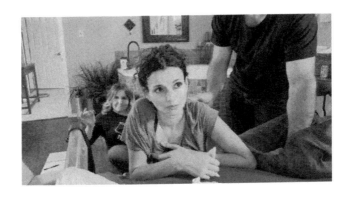

At 10 cm it was time to focus
my breaths downwards.

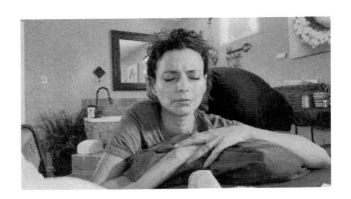

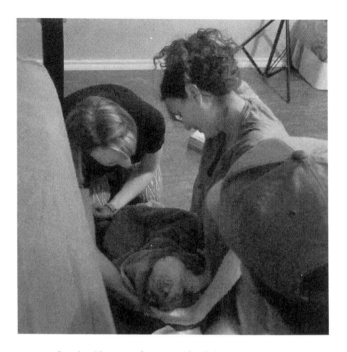

At 6:41 p.m. he made his entrance!

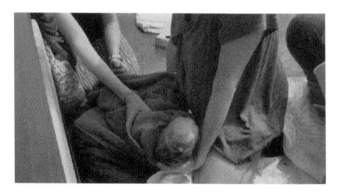

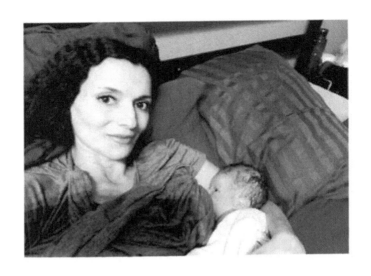

I was pretty tired,
but felt so victorious!

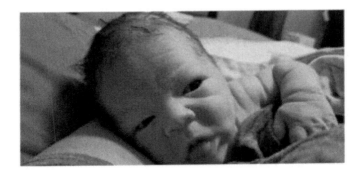

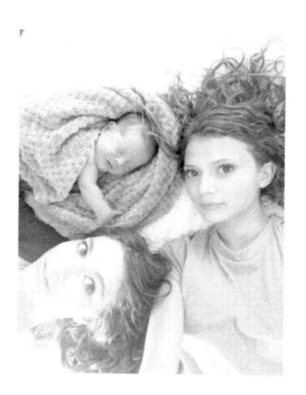

These two gals were
always by my side.

Chapter 5

"Tools" for Labor

For years I have built up a "spiritual tool belt," and now I have a "labor and delivery tool belt" as well. Here are some of my favorite tools.

1. Just Swipe!
This is going to be your most important tool.

I will not be able to emphasize this enough: when fear rushes in and says (yes fear speaks) that it's starting to hurt, SWIPE! When doubts come in like I don't know if I can do this, SWIPE! When lies come in and say, I am not sure I can push anymore, SWIPE! Just like you swipe away your phone apps easily and quickly, swipe away negative thoughts out of your mind. Yes, I said easily. It is as easy as just doing it!

2. Replace!

If you are going to be doing a lot of swiping, you are going to have to do a lot replacing. So, the process is **swipe and replace.** When you swipe away a negative thought, replace it immediately with something positive. I must be honest with you, one of the things I dreaded the most in the past was the "ring of fire." It can be an intense sensation at the perineum just as the baby crowns. In the past, it caused further fear and trepidation. However, I was so in the zone and in control that I was premeditating what would be happening. I was choosing positive responses. When I felt the baby descend and that burn, instead of panicking, I took my thoughts captive and silently told myself "the ring, there it is! It is good! My baby is coming!"

You want to know something? As soon as I was done telling myself that- it was OVER! Yes, in just seconds, it was all over!! What once caused me anguish was now replaced with happy thoughts of my baby drawing near. It worked! So, dear friend, just remember, you are trying to steer clear from adrenaline during labor. Adrenaline causes the fight-or-flight response. When our bodies are pumped up with it, we become rigid and tense. It is not a good combo during labor. Our bodies should be limber, fluid and willing. Did you hear that? We should be limber- that means relaxed.

When we submit to the process, our body creates more oxytocin, rather than adrenaline. Oxytocin has been called "the cuddle hormone" and even "the love hormone." It is a labor helper because it stimulates the uterus to contract. It also has connections to breastfeeding and bonding. So, surely, we want to welcome oxytocin into our body and avoid adrenaline which counters it. Remember, every time you let fear enter in you are permitting a release of adrenaline that can slow down the process and promote pain. Replace fear with faith. There is a stress relief visual exercise I have been doing for months, and I did it on my delivery day. I visualized three pesky passengers on a bus. I imagined pulling over and dropping off each of the passengers at the curb. Each one had a name:

fear, anxiety and overwhelmed. After I dropped those troublesome characters off, I visualized picking up some new passengers. In stepped peace, trust and tranquil. As I drove away, the atmosphere was so calm and inviting. Every time fear tried to creep in, I would say to myself, "No, you are not allowed back on!" I would then think about peace filling the bus which helped to shift my focus. I just kept doing that repeatedly as necessary. I was not ruled by the "pesky passengers."

Birthing is a beautiful process that our bodies were created to do. It is not a medical condition that necessitates fixing. Giving birth is our body's gift to humanity. When we usher in life, we are taking part in a great blessing because children are a heritage from the Lord. Since, I already mentioned that the curse is no longer placed upon on us because Christ redeemed us from it that means we can now experience the birth experience apart from the curse. How fabulous is that?

3. Positive Affirmation Cards This is similar to the replace statements, but they are geared more towards saturating your mind with positivity before and during labor. I also included encouraging Bible scriptures in my card mix.

4. Support Breathing I know there are various methods of breathing available for you to study online. For early **latent and active labor (mild to moderate/strong),** it was helpful to use common stress relief type of breathing. Tension relief breathing is when you **slowly breath in through your nose until the count of four**, then **exhaling from your mouth slowly to the count eight or at least six.** Begin this breathing exercise as soon as the surge begins until it subsides.

During surges or contractions, as I inhaled, I visualized filling up a white balloon in my belly as I sent all that wonderful oxygen to my baby.

Transitional Stage (Strong to very strong) Breathing

Breathing in this stage takes a lot of focus, and my midwife told my husband, "no matter how many children women have, they always forget how to push." So, understanding the pushing process in this last stage was important to get it done efficiently. After full dilation occurred, I was encouraged to push when I was ready- or in other words when I had the urge to push. This meant taking a deep breath in and bearing down to push. This part of pushing takes more effort than the crowning stage (when baby's head emerges) Most mamas tend to tense up and stiffen the body and push with butt muscles which I did too until I corrected myself. However, when I dropped my jaw and visualized my cervix opening like a budding rose, then things started to move in the right direction.

The focus was to keep my pelvic region open, and I literally felt the baby slide down when I got in the right position and practiced the right deep breath. I did not exhale my full breath out of my mouth. Instead, I sent it down my body, and it urged the baby down the birth canal. The key to breathing was not to let all the breath out of my mouth but to send it down towards the baby. My final breath was long, rather than short or panting. Once I felt my baby drop and slide down and crown this is where breathing changed. This was when I began to try and breathe the baby out or use my breath pressure to urge the baby down.

It wasn't about using any kind of bodily force. It was more like blowing out a candle. When you blow, you can feel the breath down in your stomach. You can practice this breath during a bowel movement. Just make sure not to hold your breath because your breaths are important for your baby to receive plenty of oxygen during this phase. Many times, the baby will crown and then go sneak back up, then slide back down with the next surge. Remaining calm and as focused as possible is important to allow your body to relax and open. In the past, it was natural for me to try and force the baby out after he crowned, but this time I knew I had to make it a slower process. Doing this allowed my body to stretch slowly. Once the baby descends and crowns it should not be a problem to get that little baby out. Many times, when pushing is extended it is because a mama is not properly pushing. It could be that she is pushing all her force out of her mouth by screaming or yelling, rather than pushing the force of the breath down and out.

When I was challenged in pushing this time around my midwife put her finger on my lower perineum and coached me to push her finger out. She was redirecting my force. Right after the redirection, I changed positions from a birthing chair to a kneeling and leaning back, squatting position. All the sudden it was like BINGO! I chose the right position and the baby descended so quickly that my husband didn't even realize the baby was out! He was already halfway out before my midwife asked if he was going to catch him! Finding the best position and practicing focused breathing was definitely the best method for this phase of labor.

5. Set the Stage: Calming Atmosphere

When setting the stage for your labor space think about your five senses: sight, smell, sound, touch, taste.

1. **Sight**: Surround yourself with visuals that will empower and encourage you. My birthing center was already set up with affirmation cards on the wall which was nice. I also I laid my cards on the bed, so I could easily view them as I was hanging on the side of the bed during the last stage of labor. Some women enjoy flickering candles and find the lighting soothing. I had a diffuser on a candle flicker mode.

2. **Smell**: I suggest only natural fragrances rather than synthetics. During labor, it is possible to have a heightened sense of smell so bring items that you feel will add to the ambiance of the room. I brought a diffuser that lights up and filled the air with Rosemary essential oil which I

love! Not only did I have it in my (diffuser,) *lavender* but I put some on a cloth to smell because it is invigorating. I chose it because it is a very comforting scent that brings back happy feelings from my youth plus it is labor support oil. If you are experiencing high blood pressure, I would choose a different oil. During a rough patch of transition when I was feeling tired, my husband handed me the rosemary cloth and I remember smiling because the scent was so soothing to me. Another time I went through a brief period where I began to experience my stomach turning. At that point, I asked for my cloth with peppermint essential oil on it, and that took care of things quick. No more icky feelings.

3. **Sound:** This area was so super important to me. I brought in audio that I listened to nightly before the baby was born. It is was a positive affirmation selection. It really helped to keep me in the zone as I focused on the words. I would listen and just let it soak in. I listened to it so much I could repeat the phrases to myself even if

the audio was turned off. You can find the audio links in the index.

4. **Touch:** Thing of this section in terms of feel. For me, this meant bringing my own pillow. It was a good call because having a comfy pillow was important to me. I also brought slippers because I do not like to walk barefoot on the floor. For you, it may be soft PJs or a cuddly robe.

5. **Taste:** Whenever I am in latent labor, I always enjoy drinking orange juice. So, we brought small cans of juice that would easily fit into our bags. My daughter also pre-made some crepes for me to eat right after labor because I do not like to eat much before labor to keep my bowel empty as empty as possible. As soon as I had the baby, I was immediately totally drained, but as soon as I ate those grain-free crepes, I was sitting up and vibrant within 20 minutes after birth. This is a time to celebrate so you may even want to bring in some sparkling grape juice.

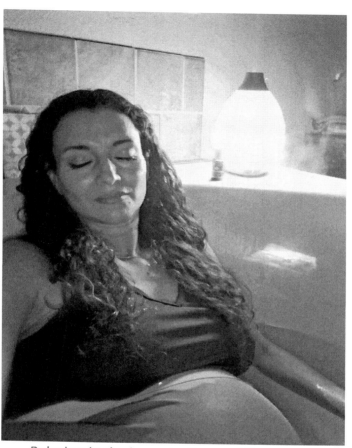

Relaxing in the jacuzzi with my diffuser near.

Chapter 6

The Essentials

The following items are on my "must-have essentials" list to include in your labor bag and for post care. (*This list does not include toiletries, clothing, baby items, etc.*)

Essential oils are a big part of my daily life, and I couldn't imagine laboring without them on the big day! Essential oils are not only soothing and beneficial for bodily support, but they can also encourage labor. It was a little piece of heaven to take a hot bath with Epsom salt and rosemary essential oil for me post birth.

Essential Oils for labor and post-care:

Make sure to check with your midwife or doctor before following any new protocol, especially during labor. I was experiencing low blood pressure the entire month before my labor, so I was freely using rosemary EO after 37 weeks and during my delivery. Note: this EO should be avoided if you are experiencing high blood pressure.

I really love citrus essential oils like lemon, lime, bergamot and grapefruit. I use vitality oils to flavor my water beautifully while providing body system support and decrease tension. Grapefruit essential oil is also helpful for post labor weight loss support. Many parents have anointed their newborns with diluted frankincense oil. Always dilute essential oils when using them on babies. I typically use **one drop of baby safe essential oil** to one roller ball of carrier oil for my infants. The safest place to use E.O.s on children is on the bottom of their feet. Remember, not all essential oils are equal in quality and purity. So, choose only high-quality therapeutic grade oils. Store EO's can be toxic if taken internally so always read labels. You can find more info on my blog.

OIL	BENEFIT	HOW TO USE
Lavender	Calming/relaxing	Inhale, Diffuse, topical
Frankincense	Skin support, tension & umbilical cord care	Rub on wrists, belly, and back
Helichrysum	Skin & Post labor support	Dilute and rub on belly and perineum. I used this right after delivery to help support normal bleeding.
Rose	Comfort and tension, possible labor progression	Diffuse, topical, inhale
Neroli	May reduce fear and tension	Inhale, diffuse
Peppermint	Reduce icky feeling, energizer, muscle tension	Inhale on a cloth, rub on lower back, dab on neck or temples.
Cypress	My go-to EO for muscle ease and tension.	Rub on tense, pulling areas
Geranium	Post care, uterine + skin support	Rub on belly, diffuse, skin care
Rosemary	Labor support, invigorating	Diffuse, Dilute topical rub (avoid if you have high blood pressure)

Supplements and Snacks

A. Primrose capsules. My midwife had me insert three capsules to help things get softened up. Note: that women with hypotension should seek professional advice before use because primrose oil can lower blood pressure.

B. WishGarden AfterEase tincture- *"lovingly formulated by the wise women at WishGarden to soothe normal and temporary afterbirth contractions."* A friend of mine gave me this tincture just before labor. I put into my labor bag and forgot about it. After I gave birth, I started to have uterine contractions. When I asked my midwife about how to handle them, she mentioned a tincture she wishes she had on hand. When she mentioned it, I remembered the gift. I had my daughter go and retrieve it, and to my delight, it was the tincture my midwife was talking about! I was relieved. I was so pleased that it went to work right away. I took it about every 30 minutes in orange juice. In the past I would take prescription strength Tylenol, but not this time. It helped with cramping and my by bleeding was the lightest it has ever been after taking it regularly the first twenty-four hours. For me, it was a must.

C. Drinks and snacks- I mentioned I brought mini oj cans. I also brought raspberry leaf too which is excellent for labor and post-delivery care. Don't forget snacks for partners as well.

D. Floradix iron liquid supplement- This gentle iron formula was so important for me after giving birth to get my iron level back up.

E. Ningxia Red packets- Liquid supplement. I took this my entire pregnancy, and my midwife said my placenta was very healthy.

F. Progesterone- Post pregnancy it is good to have a quality progesterone cream. Post pregnancy hormones can greatly fluctuate, and some women experience estrogen dominance which can cause huge mood swings and anxiety. Taking progesterone can help balance hormones. After birth, many women experience baby blues. However, I felt very moody, rather than down, and I had severe P.M.S. type symptoms. So, I

keep in mind

started using progesterone twice daily, and within two days I felt like a new happy woman.

G. Depends adult diapers- These are great for immediate post care. They don't leak like normal pads do. They are not glamorous, but they are helpful. I'm glad I brought them.

H. Lansinoh Lanolin ointment- This will help keep your breast from getting dried and cracked.

I. 12 oz Squeeze bottle to fill with water for perineum care. Add two tablespoons of vinegar to the squeeze bottle. To use: Saturate a cotton ball with the solution to keep breast clean between feedings to avoid breast yeast infections. Another way to avoid them is by combining coconut oil with a 1/8 tsp of baby probiotics and applying it to the nipple area after nursing. There is no need to wash-off breast, just gently wipe off before nursing. Follow with applying Lanolin ointment over nipple area to prevent cracking. This regimen really helped my breasts to heal quicker.

Chapter 7

Supernatural Focus

When I went into the birthing center, I came with plenty of tools. One of the most important tools for me was bringing in my full faith. I strongly believe that words are powerful and can usher in blessings or curses- aka crisis.

There is power in the tongue. I purposed to choose blessings, and I spoke them softly out loud. I chose to ignore lies and to cast away fear because **the opposite of fear is faith.** I made sure to cling to written truths of scripture. *You can find personal faith affirmations in the index.

Knowing who I am in Christ also brought me great strength and comfort during labor. When I turned my focus from guilt and shame to Christ's act of redemption on my behalf, I was able to fully receive that birth could indeed be a joyful experience. This also meant I needed to let go of past trauma: rejecting it and renouncing it. I had to be willing to trash and purge it. Along with it, I had to totally forgive past issues that happened between my husband and me. In the past, he made some crude jokes about me during labor that previously damaged my morale and could have made me feel further embarrassed during birth.

In marriage, there will be areas of disconnect. My husband did the best he knew how to during go-time. However, I had to erase the fact that we didn't really have a close connection during my past labor experiences. I needed to give him a clean slate. This was not going to be business as usual. If you really desire a supernatural labor experience you must **put away stinking thinking** because there is no room for it in a glory filled place. As I mentioned before I had plenty of tools to help me keep focused. They were simple things like breathing, essential oils, positive affirmations and a better understanding of what my body was trying to communicate to me during the process. One of my tools was worship music.

As I was bouncing on the birth ball, I can remember asking my daughter to turn on some praise music. She flipped through some songs on the phone, and as soon as Unstoppable Love by Kim Walker began playing, my eyes brimmed with tears of joy. It was such a sweet, glory-filled moment and everyone in the labor room could feel the presence of the Almighty.

No sin, no shame.
No past, no pain.
Can separate me from Your love.
No height, no depth.
No fear, no death.
Can separate me from Your love.

At that moment it was as if heaven was touching the earth. I felt all of God's goodness and mercy showering over me. I was totally present and in touch with my creator. I felt His presence in a real way, and all the glory left no room for darkness. I was completely ready to have a supernatural childbirth. I was primed to trust and have a supernatural focus which helped to create an amazing experience.

Are you ready to put away past hurts and trauma for something better? Take some time to release it all. Let it go for good. If you want a new experience, you will have to let go of the old ones completely. What is stopping you? Believe me, it's worth it!

Chapter 8

Birthing Partner's Role

The subject of birthing partners is a very important aspect of the labor process. It's not the most important part, but it can be an integral one. A birth partner can be your spouse, mother, friend or anyone you have with you as an assistant. My husband was present for all my labors, but I can't say that I felt a tight bond with him during my past births. I was glad he was there, but I always put a greater emphasis on my midwife or even my daughter as being my helper. I think he felt unsure of what to do and I could sense that which didn't allow me to lean on him like I would have if he were confident during my births. I was glad to have him, but he had some areas to grow in as a birth partner. When I was pregnant with my fifth baby, my daughter who was only ten years old accompanied during my stay at my midwife's rental house. It was down the street from the hospital where I would later give birth. I had forty-eight hours of painful pre-labor, and she was confident and attentive during my struggle. Most importantly she took the initiative to offer massages and relief. She did such a great job and was so comfortable with it all that she ended up studying midwifery for the next couple of years.

After having so many children, **I learned that the primary support a birthing mama can have is a positive mindset and second is the mental and physical support of a birth partner.** Birthing is a very intimate personal experience, and a woman should never feel forced to have people in her labor room that she feels will cause mental stress to the situation. The birth room should be protected, and this is where the birth partner enters the scene. For this last birth not only did I set out to become more educated, but I also invited my husband on the journey as I mentioned earlier. I handpicked videos that involved husbands that I felt mirrored what I desired from him during labor. We talked about what I found comforting about different techniques.

I also set some **personal boundaries** that were important to me because of past experiences. I asked him not to view my underside until my midwife announced the baby crowned. He honored that request which is why he didn't know the baby crowned because I was calm, and he wasn't looking! Everyone will have their own needs. Whatever they are and for whatever reason you have them, do not keep silent. Voice your request and let them be known. It took me some days to voice my boundary to my husband because it was attached to a past issue and I really didn't want to have to address it. However, I knew if I didn't it could cause some setbacks during pushing and I didn't want any hindrances. I could tell he was a little bothered by my request, but he was willing to honor it, and that was the most important thing. **Birth partners must be**

willing to honor the birthing mother's request. Labor is not the time to hold grudges or put personal needs before mama.

A birth partner's primary concerns should be that mama feels:

1) Protected

2) Supported

3) Nurtured

4) Heard

Now that order may be different for different women, but in general, those are the top priorities. A birthing mama should never feel mocked, disrespected or alienated. The birth partner is your advocate and a protector. If you know about personality colors (see appendix) I am a strong red/green, which basically means that I am typically confident, decisive and I like to be in control of my person.

So, it was no surprise to my family that I chose two midwives that are strong red personalities as well. For me, giving birth such a place of vulnerability that I felt I needed to pick strong women who would intervene on my behalf allowing me to set my guard down and trust their judgment and wisdom. I needed a liaison who would "drive" if necessary and not just go along for the ride. I felt very comfortable and confident in my pick for midwives, and that was so important to me. With that said, a situation comes to my mind as I am sharing this insight with you.

After a month of poor sleep and a baby that was so low that my body was sore, I finally arrived at the point of agreeing to encourage my labor by having my water broken. I was pretty tired, and after the quick procedure, my midwife gave me a list of things she wanted me to do to get things going, "I want you to get up and go for a walk and do the breast pump. You can also use the birth ball." I was so very tired, and I really didn't feel like doing any of it. However, I responded with a head nod and a quiet, "OK." Suddenly my birth partner/hubby spoke up and advocated for me. It was not in a confrontational way but in a supportive way. He became a voice for me. After I agreed to do what the midwife requested, he responded, "It is possible for her to take a short nap because she is pretty tired?" Of course, this was totally counter to what the midwife just asked. We were trying to get things started after all, and here he was asking if I could take a nap. Gratefully, he did ask because she paused and then said, "OK, but I want her to wake up and do all those things mentioned." For the next forty-five minutes, my husband gave me a foot and leg massage with lotion, and I fell asleep.

Although I felt no excruciating pain during labor that doesn't mean that I wasn't exhausted because I was. In the last phase I progressed quickly and had my baby just two hours after my nap. When you run a marathon it is tiring, but oh so rewarding and this was no different. I honestly, do not know if I would've had enough energy to push had I not taken that nap. When my husband spoke up for me it was a new day and a new way. He took the initiative and spoke up where I was silent to address my needs. Because he did, I felt fully supported which made for a better labor experience for me. Not only did he become a voice for me that day, but when I was fatigued and tempted to momentarily lose focus, he would pop an affirmation card with just the right saying in front of my face. I wasn't sure how the card thing was going to work. I thought he would mention some of the sayings to me throughout labor but instead, he didn't say a word. He would just pop one up in front of me, and I would take it in with relief and just smile. While I was pushing and fatigued the phone rang very loud a couple of times, and by the second ring, my husband asked for the ringer to be turned off. I was relieved. It didn't occur to me to tell my girls to turn off the ringer because I was too much in my zone, but each time the phone rang it caused static in the air and momentary stress.

The Latent Stage

The later transitional stage is where the birth partner will play the greatest roll. This is the stage where mama needs to be zeroed in and focused on what is happening to her body. **The least amount of stuff she must focus on outside herself the better**. So, the partner should be super attentive and ready to read her body signals or listen to her quiet requests. Have water ready in case she gets thirsty or ice chips if they are available. Also, have her essential oil cloths ready to go.

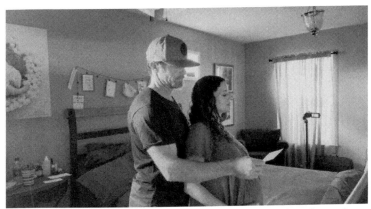

Every time I look at these images of my husband and I it evokes such a warm place of intimacy in my heart.

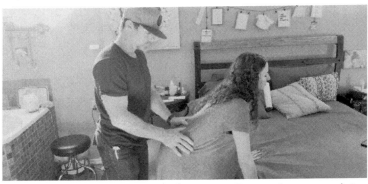

This year marks our 21st year of marriage and I can say, this year I fell head over heels in love with my husband.

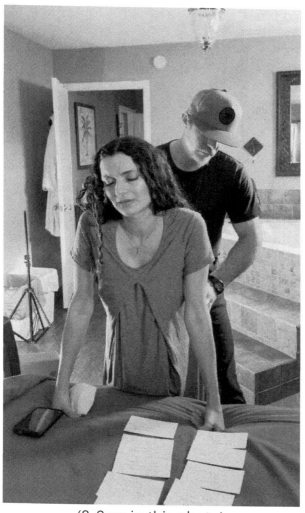

(8-9cm in this photo)

Another helpful thing my husband did was pressure point massage. He applied pressure at around BL32 acupressure site. This was so extremely helpful. This spot can be found just above the tailbone on each side of the spine where there are dimples on your lower back, you can Google to find it. Every time I had a powerful surge, I would have my partner apply very firm strong pressure until it subsided. It really helped to balance things out so that I did not experience pain.

Once upon a time, I used to think that having my husband in the room was nice, but I felt like if I had a choice of who to have with me, I would have chosen my daughter. I know that doesn't sound great, but for me, it used to be about survival and she was just so attentive. After this labor though, my husband and I found a sweet spot in the process, and it was amazing! Just two days after giving birth I did a social media post describing my initial feelings about the birth.

A big shout out to my husband. This was such a special labor and birth because we are at a different stage in our marriage and the bind was so tight this time. Not only was a baby born yesterday, but also another level in trust and commitment to each other. I know my husband saw a side of me that he has never seen before. How do I know? Because I conquered something for myself #totalControl I have never been able to pull it off to such a degree before... Complete control of my being, emotions, person, fears, and ideas. I chose truth and faith. #Empowerment

Of course, I always give thanks to Yahweh for strengthening me every step of the way. I have a new understanding of the scripture **"In quietness and in confidence is your strength."** *– Isa. 30:15*

I guess I never realized how going after a positive birth could impact my life. Initially, I was just looking for hope in the process. I wasn't aware that pursuing a positive labor experience would lead to such personal gratification and such growth in my marriage, but it did both. Usually, after labors I am not only left tired, but somewhat traumatized. **This time I was still tired, but after I got my second wind I felt like SUPERWOMAN.** I felt like I could conquer anything in life!

Are you ready to do more than just believe for a fearless childbirth?

If so, I pray that you will be more than a conqueror as you usher new life into this world!

Conquer fear.
Conquer lies.
Conquer doubts.

Boldly, go after an empowered childbirth and reach for your own **FEARLESS** testimony!

Appendix

Swipe and Replace Statements

It's going to hurt. - My body was created to birth.

It's painful. - It's a blessing.

I don't think I can push anymore - I can do this! I got this!

I don't know how to push - I am a strong woman, breath, hold, push!

I am losing control - My body knows what to do

I am too weak - I am powerful

Someone help me! - I am surrounded with support

I am scared - I was created to do this, or I am in control when I work with my body

Practical Tips:

Each replacement statement allows oxytocin to flood your body, rather than adrenaline which produces the fight or flight response. Remember that your birth partner can also read the replace statements to you if you are expressing swipe/fear statements. When you feel your body getting tense, relax your shoulders and drop them. If your partner sees your eyebrows furrowing have them lightly touch your forehead to remind you to relax your brow. You can do this!

Faith Affirmations

Who am I?

I am loved. 1 John 3:3

I am accepted. Ephesians 1:6

I am a child of God. John 1:12

I am a joint heir with Jesus, sharing His inheritance with Him. Romans 8:17

I am united with God and one spirit with Him. 1 Corinthians 6:17

I am redeemed and forgiven. Colossians 1:14

I am a new creation because I am in Christ. 2 Corinthians 5:17

I do not have a spirit of fear, but of love, power, and a sound mind. 2 Timothy 1:7

I am God's co-worker. 2 Corinthians 6:1

I have direct access to God Ephesians. 2:18

I am chosen to bear fruit John. 15:16

I can ask God for wisdom and He will give me what I need. James 1:5

Verses for Labor

Prov 31:25 Strength and honour are her clothing; and she shall rejoice in time to come.

Isa 40:31 But they that wait upon the LORD shall renew *their* strength; they shall mount up with wings as eagles; they shall run, and not be weary; *and* they shall walk, and not faint.

Philippians 4:13 I can do all things through Christ which strengtheneth me.

Psalms 127:3 Lo, children *are* an heritage of the LORD: *and* the fruit of the womb *is his* reward.

Isa 26:3 Thou wilt keep him in perfect peace, whose mind is stayed on thee; because he trusteth in thee.

Isa 40:29 He giveth power to the faint; and to them that have no might he increaseth strength.

1 sam 1:27 For this child I prayed; and the Lord hath given me my petition which I asked of him:

Isa 65:23 They shall not labour in vain, nor bring forth for trouble; for they are the seed of the blessed of the Lord, and their offspring with them.

Trust Affirmations

I trust my body.

I trust my instincts.

I trust my birth team.

Helpful Books & Resources

POSITIVE BIRTH AFFIRMATION CARDS

When I went into labor I only had hand written flash cards because we didn't have a printer available. They weren't pretty, and I even spelled a word wrong on one of the cards. This was a huge disappointment because I had a beautiful photo holding up that specific card during labor. Only later did I notice I spelled women instead of woman. It was such a bummer. So, I decided next time I would make it a priority to have some lovely pre-printed cards ready! You can find the 36 Card Set information on my blog. I also vlog there and podcast.

www.EmmaSara.com

View my birth story and more on my YouTube channel:

www.youtube.com/emmasaramcmillion

The Positive Birthing Company I found the Video Birthing Series very helpful because it dealt with body function education and provided labor tools like instructions for breathing. The best part is the information and videos are FREE!
www.youtube.com/c/thepositivebirthcompany

AUDIO

Conditioning my mind by listening to positive affirmations was extremely important. Here are my favorite resources.

CHRISTIAN HYPNOBIRTHING

www.christianhypnobirthing.com/

"The world's first Christian Hypnobirthing App. Designed to bring you empowerment throughout your pregnancy and birth."

Not only do they offer a very comforting and helpful phone app, but there is also a blog and other content tailored for mamas desiring a positive birth experience.

I really suggest the use of this app because I feel it has a strong scriptural standing and it offers a great alternative to other secular hypnobirthing apps on the market. Each audio track helps to relax you and keep you focused on God's word and the wonderful workings of your body. I would describe it more as a positive birthing app. I suggest it for every birth. I really believe listening to positive affirmations helped me to get through night surges comfortably because I had a positive outlook about what was happening to my body.

This is an excerpt from the app blog:

Why Christian Hypnobirthing works. "Yes, the breathing exercises can help you feel more relaxed and calm, and therefore your contractions can feel easier. Yes, the encouraging scriptures can help you feel empowered and to know that our Heavenly Father, Lord Jesus and the Holy Spirit are with you. Yes, the positive affirmations can help you remember that God has designed you perfectly for birth and help you feel more connected to Him and your baby. But ultimately, *Christian Hypnobirthing works because GOD IS REAL*, and it is simply a tool to help you engage with Him. By engaging with our Heavenly Father, and the power that He has given to us, birth can be a truly miraculous and spiritually empowered experience." -Tara Founder of Christian Hypnobirthing

Childbirth in the Glory- Janet Angela Mills

I used this audio with my previous childbirth. It focuses on scriptures and faith promises. This time around it was a little fast paced for this season in life, but you might find it enjoyable. Available on Amazon.

Supernatural Childbirth- Jackie Mize

This book was the catalyst that propelled me to find more answers to birthing in the glory.

Gentle Babies- By Debra Raybern

Essential Oils and Natural Remedies for Pregnancy, Childbirth, Infants and Young Children. This is a must have book resource for new mamas.

Color Personality Test

This is a quick online test that is such a valuable communication tool. Take it and learn some new things about yourself and your loved ones. Strong families know how to communicate. Focused women know their strengths and weaknesses. This is perfect tool to dig deep!

jacobadamo.com/personality-colors-quiz/

Labor Bag

- [ ] _____
- [ ] _____
- [ ] _____
- [ ] _____
- [ ] _____
- [ ] _____
- [ ] _____
- [ ] _____
- [ ] _____
- [ ] _____
- [ ] _____
- [ ] _____
- [ ] _____

Creative Corner!

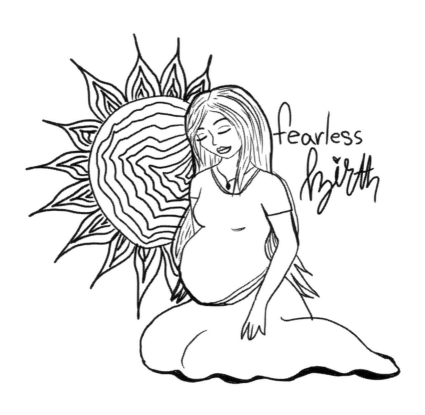

Creative Corner!

Notes

Author

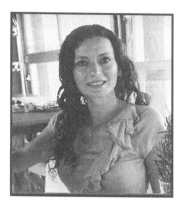

EmmaSara is a CNCH, Certified Natural Health Counselor. She has been passionately studying integrative health for 15 years. She is the founder of Fab & Fit and she enjoys teaching monthly Compelled Lifestyle workshops.

She has eight amazing children and a supportive husband. Together they are building up a dream on their 100-acre ranch in Far West Texas.

Let's connect!

Thanks for taking the time to read my book. I pray that it was a great encouragement to you. **Don't forget to leave your book review on Amazon and share the gift of HOPE with others! Let's connect on social media and tag me with a shout out!**

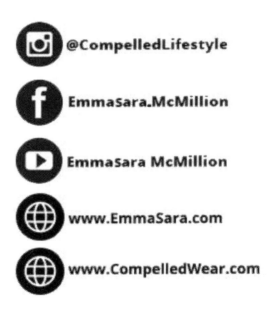

@CompelledLifestyle

EmmaSara.McMillion

EmmaSara McMillion

www.EmmaSara.com

www.CompelledWear.com

I want to see your beautiful
Fearless Birth Babies!
So, don't forget to take a photo with your
newborn and your *Fearless Birth book.*
Post it on social media using the hashtag
#EMPOWEREDfearlessbirth
I will be hosting monthly promos and giveaways
for mamas who use the hashtag!
Plus, you could be featured on
my blog and Podcast!

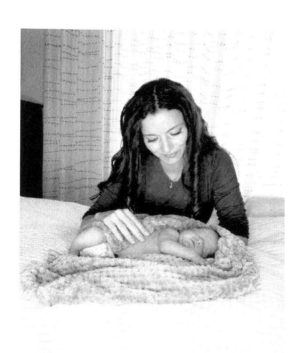

This is Your Story

Be Fearless.

Your baby is now here! It's time to capture this moment. You won't regret it! So, what's on your heart?

_____

_____

_____

_____

_____

_____

_____

_____

_____

_____

_____

_____

_____

_____

_____

_____

_____

_____

_____

Be Present. Be Gracious.

Be Joyful.

35857937R00062

Made in the USA
Middletown, DE
08 February 2019